# GETTING PREGNANT FAST

*The Essential 'How to Get Pregnant Fast Guide' that will Turn Your Dream of Having a Baby into a Reality*

## Paige Mathisen

**Copyright © 2015 by
Paige Mathisen**

All rights reserved. No part of this publication may be reproduced, distributed, or transmitted in any form or by any means, including photocopying, recording, or other electronic or mechanical methods without the prior written permission of the publisher, except in the case of brief quotations embodied in critical reviews and certain other non-commercial uses permitted by copyright law. For permission, direct requests to the publisher.

Distribution of this book without the prior permission of the author is illegal and therefore punishable by law.

Evita Publishing, PO Box 306, Station A, Vancouver Island, BC V9W 5B1 Canada

# Table of Contents

*Introduction - 5*

## Chapter 1

*Before Trying For a Baby - 9*

## Chapter 2

*A Step by Step Guide for Quick Conception - 26*

## Chapter 3

*Early Signs of Pregnancy – A Week after Conception - 53*

## Chapter 4

*The Top 15 Best Fertility Foods to Raise Your Chances of GettingPregnant Fast - 62*

## Chapter 5

*Foods to Avoid When Trying To Conceive - 71*

### **Chapter 6**

*Is It Possible To Conceive Naturally After 40? - 77*

### **Chapter 7**

*Considering Different Ways to Get Pregnant - 85*

*Conclusion - 91*

# Introduction

I know it's hard to keep believing that conception can happen for you when you're trying but not seeing the results that you desire. Don't worry, I'm living proof that getting pregnant can happen no matter how long you've been trying!

My husband and I tried to get pregnant for years. It seemed like all my friends were getting pregnant but somehow I couldn't. There were many times that I wanted to throw in the towel and call it quits but I just couldn't give up my dream of having a baby.

Desperate to increase my chances of getting pregnant, I aggressively started reading every book I could find on infertility, getting pregnant, and conception.

I applied everything I learned, from diligently calculating my ovulation and watching for fertility signs, having sex often and at specific times, eating foods that would boost my fertility as well as educating my husband on what he could do to improve our chances.

We continued to work these techniques over and over and after only a couple of months... it happened...my dream of getting pregnant became a reality at 37 years old!

Then, surprisingly, I got pregnant again a year and a half after the birth of my first child using the same techniques!!

I wrote this book specifically for you, and I know from experience that the information in this book will increase your chances of getting pregnant.

In a step by step way, *Getting Pregnant Fast* will teach you the exact methods that I used to increase my chances of getting pregnant.

This guide was written with heart from my own experience in order to help you become a first time mom.

I'm not exaggerating when I say that you really can be holding your precious little baby boy or girl in three months or less.

Thank you for allowing me to help you succeed in your efforts to get pregnant.

My greatest joy is helping others like you experience the joy of motherhood!

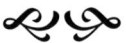

# Chapter 1

# Before Trying For a Baby

If you're like most women who have been trying to conceive without success, this is probably not the first time that you've searched out information on how to get pregnant fast. Chances are that the endless array of tips and tricks available online have only confused you further and added to your frustration.

While it is true that ovulation predictor kits, cervical mucus, basal thermometers, sex positions and other baby conceiving tips that you may have read about are all very important for conception, the most important thing is to FIRST prepare yourself both physically and psychologically so that your efforts will bear fruit.

Below are some important things you need to consider FIRST before trying for a baby.

## Have a medical checkup

See your family doctor for a medical checkup so as to rule out any medical condition that might hinder your ability to conceive. Obesity or excess weight, high blood pressure and diabetes are just some of the medical conditions that can make conception difficult or even impossible.

Your doctor will review your present health, your personal medical history, your family's medical history as well as any medications you're on. Certain medications are dangerous to take during pregnancy and some have to be changed before you try to conceive.

Having a medical checkup can insure that you have the odds in your favor for quick conception.

### Eat right

You will also need to eat right if you are to enhance your ability to conceive. Every meal and snack need to follow a healthy diet. According to high ranking nutritionists, a balanced diet is composed of the following:

Protein

Vegetables

Fruits

Whole grains

Fats

Making nutritious choices now will allow your body to have a good supply of nutrients to maintain a healthy pregnancy.

You should aim for consuming two and a half cups of vegetables every day, two cups of fruit, as well as a good amount of whole grains and high calcium foods like yogurt and milk. Also make sure that you are regularly eating protein from poultry, meats, seeds, beans, nuts, and soy products.

**Start taking folic acid**

It is important to start taking folic acid to help reduce serious birth defects that may affect the brain or spinal cord of the baby you hope to conceive. It is recommended to take 400 mcg of folic acid every day for at least a month before you try to conceive and to continue that through your first trimester.

You can purchase folic acid at your local drugstore or you can take a multivitamin that contains 400mcg of folic acid. If you opt for taking a multivitamin be careful that it doesn't contain more than the daily recommended allowance (770mcg) of vitamin A unless it is in the form of beta-carotene. Too much vitamin A can cause birth defects.

### Stop drugs and alcohol

In order to conceive, you will be required to quit smoking, drinking alcohol, and doing drugs. You will also need to advise your partner to quit as well. While it is obvious that such substances can affect your unborn baby, studies have shown that they can affect the fertility of your partner as well. Alcohol, nicotine and drugs can affect male fertility through:

Chromosomal damage

Decreased motility (sperm swimming rate)

Erectile dysfunction

Many studies have proven that smoking or taking drugs can lead to pre-mature birth, low birth weight, miscarriage and a host of other problems for your developing baby. Second hand smoke can also affect your chances of conception.

It is important to note that many drugs can remain in your system after the noticeable effects have worn off so you need to stop in plenty of time before you try to conceive.

## Attain a healthy weight

Getting your weight in check is also very important if you are to achieve conception. Studies have shown that you might conceive easier if your weight is healthy. A low or high BMI (body mass index) can make it hard for some women to conceive. If you are unsure about your BMI, your doctor can calculate it for you.

Should your doctor find that your current weight is unhealthy, you may need to gain or lose some weight so as to boost your fertility. Your healthcare provider can advise you accordingly in regards to this.

## Start exercising

If you don't have an exercise program already, create one and start following it immediately. A healthy program should include a minimum of 30 minutes of moderate exercise such as weight training, cycling, or walking at least three times a week.

To help ease your way into an exercise program, start slowly and work your way up. You may start with walking a few minutes a day or taking the stairs instead of the elevator. Soon you will have a healthy body to enhance your chances of conception.

## Avoid lubricants

Avoid using lubricants when you are trying to conceive. Although lubricants can increase your pleasure they inhibit conception by slowing the motility of the sperm in reaching the cervix. The natural acidity of the vagina will kill the sperm as they try to free themselves from the lubricant there. You should also avoid artificial lubricants like egg whites or mineral oil.

## Consult your dentist

Oral health is just as important as your physical health when preparing for pregnancy. This is because your body will begin to experience hormonal shifts as soon as you conceive. These hormonal shifts are likely to leave you vulnerable to various oral infections such as gum disease whereby you may experience tender, swollen or red gums that will bleed whenever you brush or floss.

By taking care of your oral health before pregnancy, you will greatly reduce your chances of suffering from gum disease and other oral infections later during pregnancy.

## Have your mental health analyzed by a doctor

If you are suffering from any mental disorders such as depression, you might have difficulty conceiving. Clinical depression is a disorder that will make it difficult for a mother to take care of herself, the pregnancy, and the child.

Some of the most obvious signs of clinical depression include the following:

> Loss of interest or pleasure in things you once used to enjoy

> Decreased or increased appetite

Loss of energy

Feelings of worthlessness or hopelessness

Sleeping less or sleeping more than normal

Your practitioner or healthcare provider will be able to refer you to a psychiatrist or therapist for help if you are affected by this condition.

## Avoid infections

All women are advised to avoid infections if they have intentions of getting pregnant especially those that can harm your baby. In order to do this, you may have to avoid certain foods such as cold deli meats, raw or undercooked fish or poultry, unpasteurized cheeses and other foods that are likely to harbor dangerous bacteria.

Dangerous bacteria can cause listeriosis which is a food-borne disease that has been known to cause miscarriages and still birth. You should also avoid unpasteurized juices as they also contain dangerous bacteria such as E.coli and salmonella.

In addition to this, make sure you always wash your hands thoroughly before cooking and eating. Your fridge should also be set between 2-4 degrees Celsius and -18 degrees Celsius for your freezer. This will keep your cold foods healthy and free from harmful bacteria and spoilage.

You should also try to always wear gloves whenever you are gardening so as to avoid getting infected with toxoplasmosis which is another deadly infection that can affect your developing baby negatively. In fact, you'd probably be better off hiring someone else to do your gardening in order to reduce the risk further.

Lastly, get a flu shot or vaccine. This will lower your chances of contracting the flu virus when you get pregnant. The flu can lead to pre-term labor and pneumonia.

## Decrease any environmental risks

While it is understandable that you might not be able to handle every environmental danger around you, you should try your best to avoid most of them. For example, a job that exposes you to radiation or chemicals might be hazardous to your unborn baby once you conceive and you might have to make some changes before you start trying for a baby.

In addition to that, you might have to avoid some cleaning products, solvents and pesticides. Talking to your healthcare provider about your environment will help you determine the necessary protective measures.

**Think twice before trying for a baby**

Before deciding to have a baby, realize that once born, your baby will be your lifetime responsibility. Therefore, make sure that you are ready to shoulder this responsibility the whole way.

Ask yourself the following questions:

Are you and your partner both committed to being parents?

Are you willing to care for a baby if he or she happens to be a "special" baby or a baby born with defects or disabilities?

How will you handle childcare and work responsibilities?

Can you handle the cost involved in raising kids?

How will you and your partner raise your children on a spiritual level, if you have differences in this area?

**Stop birth control**

After you are absolutely sure that you want a baby, stop birth control. Don't panic if you find that you still haven't conceived immediately after stopping birth control. Relax and give your body time because there are some forms of birth control that will have a more lasting effect when compared to others.

According to experts at the American College of Obstetrics and Gynecology, if you are on birth control pills, you need to continue taking them until your current cycle ends, after which you can stop taking them the next month and start trying for a baby then.

Other experts will recommend that you wait for one month or more after stopping the pills before expecting results. For example, the manufacturers of Depo-Provera say that it takes twelve weeks (three months or so) for the contraceptive hormone to leave the body of the user.

On the other hand, Norplant manufacturers claim that it only takes three days for the effects to wear off after the sticks have been removed.

If you are using condoms, a diaphragm, or a cervical cap, you may achieve quicker results because there is no delay in seeing results with these. You just remove them and your possibility of conceiving is immediate.

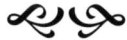

# Chapter 2

# A Step by Step Guide for Quick Conception

## Step 1

### Identify your fertile days

Your most fertile days are when you are ovulating. So, what is ovulation?

Every month, about twenty eggs mature inside your ovaries. Ovulation is when the ripest, mature egg is released from an ovary and travels into the fallopian tube. The egg then waits in the fallopian tube for sperm to arrive and fertilize it.

During sexual intercourse sperm are deposited in the vagina. 99% of those sperm either leak out of the vagina or die in the acidic environment of the vagina. Any sperm that reach the cervix are able to survive there due to the cervical mucus that helps keep them alive. Once the sperm travels through the cervical mucus and reaches the uterine cavity it has a chance of reaching the egg in the fallopian tube.

If the mature egg is fertilized by sperm it travels down the fallopian tube and implants itself in the uterine cavity. The lining of the uterus becomes thicker in order to prepare for the fertilized egg. The fertilized embryo then begins to grow in the uterus for the next nine months.

If conception does not occur then the uterine lining along with blood will be shed. When the shedding of the uterine lining and the fertilized egg occurs it is called menstruation.

The egg released into your fallopian tube lives between twelve to twenty-four hours after you've ovulated. The egg and the sperm have to collide and fertilize within this time.

Sperm can live in your body for seven days. This is good news because it gives you about six fertile days when you can conceive.

If you have sex during this fertile time, your ovulated egg is likely to meet healthy sperm waiting to fertilize it in the fallopian tube.

## Four methods that will help you identify your fertile days

### Method #1

### Calculate your ovulation

The best way to calculate your most fertile time is to buy a calendar and keep track of your cycles.

Record the first day of your cycle. The first day of your cycle is the first day of your period. Also record the amount of days in your cycle.

In recording this, make sure you understand that your personal menstrual cycle begins on the first day of your period and ends on the last day before you start your period again. It is recommended to keep track of your cycle for three to four months.

As you track your menstrual cycle you will notice that it can vary per month. That's okay. Simply average the length of your cycle over a three to four month span.

Ovulation normally occurs fourteen days before the beginning of a menstrual cycle. To estimate when you are likely to be ovulating, just subtract fourteen days from the length of your cycle.

Women have different cycles and it is therefore important to determine your individual cycle.

If your cycle is twenty eight days, you will most likely ovulate around the fourteenth day.

If your cycle is thirty five days, you are likely to ovulate around the twenty first day.

There are ovulation calculators available online to track this if you'd like to go that route.

Just remember that any kind of ovulation calculation only provides an estimate of your ovulation date.

If your menstrual cycle varies per month, it can be difficult to predict your actual ovulation date. A fertility doctor can provide various tests that can help you get a more accurate prediction.

Though this might be a little more accurate, learning to recognize your own body's fertility signs can help a lot.

# Method #2

# How to recognize your body's fertility signs

If you are in tune with your body you will be able to recognize certain fertility signs that it might be showing you.

Below is a list of signs that your body gives you to tell you that you are ovulating.

## Cervical mucus

Cervical mucus is discharge that you see on your underwear or toilet paper when you go to the bathroom. If you are sensitive to what your cervical mucus looks like, you can determine when you are fertile. Here's what you can expect through your cycle.

During your period you will of course have menstrual blood. When your period ends you will be dry and clear for a while. After that, your cervical mucus discharge will be cloudy and have a consistency that is similar to sticky rice. These are not prime fertile days.

As you get closer to ovulation, usually a few days ahead, the mucus will increase and change in texture. This change means that the hormone oestrogen is increasing in your body. This is a sign that you are close to ovulating. You will know when you are most fertile when your mucus becomes slippery, thin, clear, stretchy, and similar to raw egg whites. The last day that you see this mucus indicates your most fertile day. This usually occurs the day before or day of ovulation.

The best time to check your cervical mucus is in the morning. Some women have enough discharge that they can check their cervical mucus on their toilet paper after they wipe. Other women have to sit on the toilet and insert their index or middle finger into their vagina, reach toward their cervix then examine their mucus that way.

The body produces cervical mucus to make it easier for the sperm to swim all the way up through to the uterus. It nourishes the sperm and enables it to survive in a woman's body longer so that it has more of a chance of meeting the egg in the fallopian tube.

### Pain in your belly

Some women can feel something going on in their ovaries around ovulation. This can vary from a mild achy feeling, spurts of pain, a one-sided back ache or abdominal pain or tenderness. If you feel pain like this around the same time each month, check your cervical mucus. Pain can be a good indicator of ovulation.

### Sore breasts

Higher levels of oestrogen before ovulation can make your breasts feel sore, tender or tingly. Being sensitive to this is a good way of recognizing that you are nearing ovulation.

### You feel sexy

If you notice a rise in your sexual desire and you feel more sexy and flirty, this may be a sign that you are most fertile.

Medical evidence has proven that as you near ovulation you will feel more attractive and even unconsciously choose clothes that flatter you. This in turn will make you more attractive to others. You will also naturally smell good at this time. Your body odor is more sexy to men when you are most fertile.

**Your cervix will be higher**

If you are engaging in more invasive testing to check your fertility, you can test your cervix to see how high it is in your vagina. When you ovulate, the cervix drops. This is a more sensitive way of testing fertility because you really need to know your body in order to determine this.

## Method #3

## Basal body temperature charting

For centuries women have identified their fertile days by tracking their body temperatures (basal body temperature charting) immediately after waking up in the morning or after at least three to five hours of uninterrupted sleep.

This is another way that your body tells you that you might be ovulating. Changes in your body temperature may indicate ovulation.

Your basal body temperature is your lowest body temperature within a twenty four hour period of time. It is recommended to track your body temperature in the morning when you are fully rested.

Upon waking in the morning put a basal thermometer (available at your local drugstore) in your mouth to check your temperature. It is important to note that you can't get up out of bed to go get your thermometer or do anything else until you've taken your temperature. Consider putting an alarm under your pillow so that you engage in the least amount of movement as possible.

Unlike a regular thermometer, the basal thermometer tracks extremely small incremental degree changes. You can take your temperature orally, vaginally, or rectally. Any method is fine. Just make sure to stick with the same method all the time and take your temperature at about the same time every day.

When you purchase a basal thermometer it will come with a temperature plotting chart. You can also print a basal body temperature chart online as well. A temperature plotting chart is important because it will allow you to track your temperature for a cycle or two so that you can see what your ovulation pattern is.

Before you ovulate, your basal body temperature will range from 97.2 to 97.7 degrees Fahrenheit. Two or three days AFTER you ovulate you will notice a rise in your body temperature of 0.4 to 1.0 degree which continues until your next period. It is possible that your temperature might spike occasionally but unless it stays up consistently, you haven't ovulated yet.

A basal body temperature (BBT) chart will only tell you that you've already ovulated. Tracking the first month therefore won't help you much, but tracking your BBT for a few months will allow you to see a pattern in your cycle and therefore predict ovulation.

## How to use the basal body temperature chart

Typically a basal body temperature chart will say "Cycle day" at the top. The first day of your cycle is the day that you get your period. Fill in that date. Continue to fill in the days of the week that correspond to your cycle.

Take your basal body temperature every day and check your cervical mucus as well. With a dot, indicate your temperature on the chart. Also, make a note of what your cervical mucus looks like under "CM type" typically at the bottom of your chart. If you connect the dots you can see fluctuations in your body temperature from day to day.

Near the end of your cycle, go back over your chart and look for the day that you ovulated. It is normally the last day that your cervical mucus resembled raw egg whites, or the day after that followed by two to three days of a consistent rise in temperature. Highlight that day and make a note of which cycle day it fell on.

For your next cycle, use a new chart to see if you ovulate on the same cycle day. Continue this charting approach for a few months. It should enable you to predict when you ovulate in your cycle.

If your ovulation day is the same from month to month, plan to have sex on that day and on the surrounding days. If your ovulation day varies, look for other patterns that can help you predict your ovulation day. One example might be that when you are on the verge of ovulating, you have two to three days where your cervical mucus is like raw egg whites, then it might dip before rising the next day. Not every woman is the same so it's important to be in tune with your own body to predict ovulation as best as you can.

Have sex every day or every other day during your most fertile period. This is always a good way to cover your bases and give yourself the best chance of fertilization.

## Method #4

## Ovulation prediction kits

Ovulation prediction kits or OPKs alert women when the egg is about to be released, which enables them to have sex BEFORE and NOT after the egg has been released.

To be able to detect when the egg is about to be released, OPKs will first detect a surge or swell in the LH (luteinizing hormone) in the urine. This normally occurs thirty six to forty eight hours before ovulation.

There are two types of OPKs available on the market today. The first is recommended for women who have extremely regular cycles. These women have a rough idea of when ovulation is likely to occur because their cycles are so regular. That knowledge allows them to begin using the kit beforehand; usually around the week they expect to ovulate.

The other type of OPK is for everyday use and it is recommended for women whose cycles are unpredictable or less regular. These OPK's are slightly more expensive than the ones mentioned above but they are very important to have in order to predict ones ovulation period.

## Step 2

### Have sex often

In order to get pregnant, sperm has to fertilize the egg. It makes sense then that in order to increase your chances of getting pregnant you should constantly allow sperm to be ready and available to fertilize the egg. Having regular sex, at least every two to three days, keeps sperm hovering in the fallopian tubes and increases your chances of conceiving. Having sex when your cervical mucus is slippery and most receptive to sperm will also increase your odds of getting pregnant.

Your most fertile days are usually three days before your ovulation period through to when you actually ovulate. This is the best time for sex, however, starting earlier won't hurt. In fact, there are women who have conceived almost six days prior to when they ovulated.

Going for a long time without having sex will cause a build up of dead sperm in your partner's semen which won't get you pregnant. You are therefore advised to have sex at least once before your fertile days in order to get rid of any dead sperm.

Some good advice you can give your partner is to wear loose underwear or pants. This is because some studies have suggested that sperm count can drop drastically when testicles are overheated or constricted. Avoiding saunas, hot tubs, and extreme exercises is also a good idea.

In order to ensure that sperm is healthy, plentiful, and strong, your partner can also do the following.

## Avoid or reduce alcohol consumption

Studies have shown that daily alcohol consumption can decrease sperm count and testosterone levels, and encourage the production of abnormal sperm.

## Avoid tobacco and other recreational drugs

This has also been identified to cause reduced sperm function.

## Consume enough key nutrients

Calcium, folic acid, zinc, and vitamins C and D play an

important role in promoting the creation of strong, plentiful, and wiggly sperm.

Note that the sooner your partner begins to work on creating healthier sperm, the sooner you are likely to conceive. In most cases, it will take up to three months for him to develop healthy sperm after making the necessary adjustments.

## Step 3

## Have sex the old fashioned way

Studies have proven that having sex the old fashioned way (missionary position) can enhance your chances of conceiving. According to these studies, when a woman lies on her back after sex, it prevents sperm from leaking out. This ensures that the sperm will travel all the way to the fallopian tube to meet the egg.

One particular study that took place in Amsterdam showed that women who lie flat on their backs for a minimum of fifteen minutes after being artificially inseminated were 50% more likely to conceive when compared to women who got up immediately after the procedure.

## Step 4

### Relax and enjoy the process

In most cases, women who are desperate, or in a hurry to become pregnant, often feel anxious or even depressed about it. While this is understandable, a woman who is not stressed is more likely to conceive than a stressed or depressed woman.

This is because the hypothalamus (a gland in the brain that controls the process of ovulation) does not work efficiently under stress. Ovulation therefore, is either delayed or ceases to occur during a cycle due to the stress.

It is therefore advised to do all you can to relax and enjoy the process of getting pregnant. Most importantly avoid the "must get pregnant this time" trap. Know that this will only be detrimental in achieving your goal of conception.

## Step 5

## Prepare to test

After making love, you will probably be extremely anxious to test. The earlier you realize that you are pregnant, the better it will be for your health and the health of your developing baby. This is because you will not only start prenatal quite early, you will also start taking care of yourself more by eating and drinking healthy foods.

There are some home testing kits that will enable you to start testing as early as ten days after ovulation. However, experts recommend that you wait at least until a few days after a missed period for a more accurate result. Testing too early can give you a false negative when you are actually pregnant.

In such cases, your body might not be producing enough pregnancy hormones to be dctected by your testing kit. The best time to test is a few days after you have missed your period because by this time your body will have produced enough hCG hormones for easy detection. Performing a home pregnancy test or getting one done by your doctor is the most reliable sign of pregnancy.

## What if the test is negative?

If the test is negative, there's no need to panic. Many couples don't succeed until they have tried to conceive several times. In fact, studies have shown that more than half of the couples trying to conceive get positive results by the 3$^{rd}$ month, while 85% will succeed within the first year. In most cases, women miscalculate their most fertile days or their partner's sperm never gets the chance to fertilize their egg.

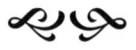

# Chapter 3

# Early Signs of Pregnancy - A Week after Conception

For many women, signs of pregnancy will not appear for weeks. There are other women however, who will experience a few signs as soon as one week after conception.

If you are among this fortunate group, you are likely to notice the following:

### Implantation bleeding

Implantation bleeding occurs when the fertilized egg attaches itself to the uterine lining. When this occurs, a tiny amount of blood may be shed. This normally happens around one week after a woman has conceived and is usually the first sign of pregnancy for most women. This kind of bleeding is usually very light and will only last for one to two days. It is also lighter in color when compared to regular menstrual flow. It can either be pink, red or brown and may be accompanied by slight cramping.

## Fatigue

A few moments after the fertilized egg has implanted itself into the wall of your uterus, pregnancy hormones will be released. The release of these hormones can trigger extreme feelings of tiredness or fatigue. In addition to this, increased blood production, low blood pressure, and low blood sugar can occur during early pregnancy. This can also likely cause fatigue or tiredness.

## Headaches

Hormone surges and increased blood circulation that are normally caused by the implantation of the fertilized egg into the uterus wall can cause you to experience headaches. While these headaches can occur only during early pregnancy, they may persist throughout the entire pregnancy for some women.

## Breast changes and soreness

For some women, breasts can change as soon as one week after conceiving. In fact, sensitive, sore breasts caused by rising hormone levels are one of the earliest signs of pregnancy. The soreness may resemble the soreness you feel in your breasts just before a period, only this soreness is like a double version of that. Other changing breast symptoms can include swollen, larger than normal, tender or tingly breasts. The nipples might also become more erect, darker or larger. The discomfort that you feel in your breasts should decrease after the first trimester when your body has adjusted to the hormonal changes.

**Delayed menstruation**

The most common sign of pregnancy is a missed period. However, this is usually not a clear indication of pregnancy because a missed period can occur as a result of various conditions and circumstances with pregnancy being one of them. Typically, seven out of ten women experience pregnancy symptoms two weeks after their missed period.

## Food cravings and an altered sense of smell

Food cravings are also a well know sign of possible pregnancy. Just the smell of certain foods can make you feel nauseous. You might also start loathing some foods and craving others. For some women, these symptoms can occur even before they have missed their period. It is also common to experience a metallic taste in your mouth or find that you have an aversion to certain aromas of foods that you once enjoyed.

## A need to pass urine more frequently

This usually occurs around six weeks into your first trimester. After you get pregnant, hormonal changes cause blood to flow at a more rapid rate through your kidneys. This causes the bladder to fill more often. During the course of your pregnancy, your body produces up to fifty percent more blood than it did before you got pregnant. This causes extra fluid to get processed through your kidneys which in turn means your bladder will become full more often. Should you notice a burning sensation or pain when passing urine during this time, it could be a urinary tract infection and you should seek treatment immediately.

## Nausea

Nausea is often referred to as "morning sickness" though it can happen at any time of the day. This condition affects seventy five percent of pregnant women during the first trimester. It typically begins two weeks after a missed period. The symptoms include vomiting and/or queasiness. Morning sickness often ends after fourteen weeks into the pregnancy though some women experience it for another month after that. It is also common for some women to experience nausea later in their pregnancy while other women continually experience morning sickness throughout their pregnancy.

## Mood swings

Some women experience an extreme case of good and bad emotions. It is also common for depression and anxiety to increase. This happens because the neurotransmitter levels in the brain are affected by the hormonal shifts that happen during pregnancy. Your healthcare provider should be able to offer advice on coping with this condition so that it doesn't affect your developing baby in a negative way.

## Bloating

The hormonal changes that occur during pregnancy can cause bloating. This can make your waistline expand thus making it harder to fit into your clothes.

## Your basal body temperature stays high

If you have been charting your basal body temperature and notice that it stays high for eighteen days in a row, that is a good sign that you're probably pregnant.

## A positive home pregnancy test

Most home pregnancy tests are not sensitive enough to detect pregnancy until a week after a missed period. A baby starts developing inside of you before you can tell that you're pregnant so it's important to take care of your health while you're waiting to find out if you're pregnant.

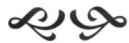

# Chapter 4

# The Top 15 Best Fertility Foods to Raise Your Chances of Getting Pregnant Fast

You may have heard that some foods can enhance your fertility. This is absolutely correct! Food and fertility are naturally linked together so getting the right balance of vitamins and minerals is essential when you are trying to conceive. Here is a list of fertility-boosting super foods for a healthy reproductive system.

## Beans

Various studies have identified beans as a fertility booster. These studies discovered that conception was likely to occur in a woman who constantly ingested both animal and plant-based proteins. Beans are an excellent source of plant protein. Lentils, nuts, and tofu are great as well!

## Ice cream

Studies have shown that having one to two daily servings of whole milk or milk products such as ice cream, can help protect against ovulatory infertility. On the contrary, low-fat milk and skim milk have been identified to hinder ovulation. In spite of this, do not go overboard. One or two servings is enough.

## Leafy vegetables

Romaine, arugula, spinach, broccoli and all other dark, leafy greens are rich sources of folate which is a well known ovulation enhancer. Make sure to have your partner consume these vegetables too for healthier sperm. Broccoli in particular, contains high levels of phytosterols which support the hormone system in women that are trying to conceive. Phytosterols are also important in preventing oestrogen overload. This condition however is more common for women in their mid-thirties and older.

## Pumpkin seeds

Pumpkin seeds are a high source of non-heme iron. Non-heme iron is found in iron-fortified foods and certain plants. One particular study discovered that women who regularly take non-heme iron supplements have a higher chance of conceiving than women who don't. A good way to prepare pumpkin seeds is to toast them in the oven for a crispy snack.

## Whole wheat bread

Consuming whole wheat bread and other unrefined products will likely boost your fertility because these are rich sources of complex carbohydrates which take longer to digest. This allows your insulin/blood sugar levels to remain stable. High levels of insulin are known to negatively affect reproductive hormones and significantly disrupt conception efforts.

## Olive oil

Olive oil is a type of monounsaturated fat that can increase insulin sensitivity and reduce inflammation in the body. Inflammation has been known to hinder ovulation and conception. It has also been known to interfere with the early development of the embryo.

## Wild salmon

Wild salmon is very rich in omega-3 fatty acids which can help regulate reproductive hormones and increase blood flow towards the reproductive organs. Omega-3 fats are also believed to reduce the possibility of miscarriage because they control the majority of the body's inflammatory response. When there is excessive inflammation in the body it over stimulates the immune response and this can lead to miscarriage. Oily fish like salmon also help to regulate sex gland functioning. Salmon also has a lower mercury content when compared to other fatty fish. Fish that are high in mercury content should be avoided entirely when trying to conceive.

## Bananas

Bananas contain vitamin B6. This is one of the most vital vitamins when it comes to conception because vitamin B6 helps to regulate your hormones. If you are deficient in vitamin B6 it can cause poor egg and sperm development

## Asparagus

Asparagus contains Folic Acid. Folic acid supplements are recommended when trying to conceive, so getting some folic acid in your foods can harness the power of this magic nutrient even faster. Studies have also found that folic acid can reduce the risk of ovulatory failure.

## Sunflower seeds

Sunflower seeds are packed with zinc which is a vital nutrient for both female and male fertility.

Zinc is also full of protein which is an important nutrient for a fertility diet.

## Shellfish

The magic nutrient in shellfish is vitamin B12. Studies have shown a correlation with B12 deficiency and abnormal oestrogen levels.

This can cause an interference with the implantation of the fertilized egg.

B12 also strengthens the endometrial lining in egg fertilization thus decreasing the chances of miscarriage.

## Almonds

Almonds contain vitamin E that has been known to improve sperm health in men. It is also an antioxidant that can protect the egg and sperm DNA.

## Citrus fruits

Citrus fruits contain vitamin C. For women, vitamin C has been known to improve hormonal balance. For men, studies have shown that vitamin C can improve sperm count and sperm motility (the sperms ability to properly move toward the egg).

## Tofu

The important ingredient in Tofu that promotes conception is iron. Studies have shown that women deficient in iron have suffered from a lack of ovulation. Iron deficiency was potentially responsible for poor egg health as well.

## Wild Yams

Experts believe that the starch in wild yams helps to stimulate ovulation. Studies have found that twins are common in cultures where the women's intake of yams was higher than other cultures.

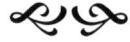

# Chapter 5

# Foods to Avoid When Trying To Conceive

Just as there are foods that can help boost your fertility there are also foods that you shouldn't eat when you are trying to conceive. This chapter outlines foods to stay away from and why.

### Peas

Peas are great because they contain a natural chemical known as m-xylohydroquinone which might hinder your efforts to conceive. In fact, some studies are underway on how peas can potentially be used as a natural contraceptive.

## Unpasteurized Dairy Foods

Cheese and milk that haven't been pasteurized can contain dangerous bacteria that can harm your conception efforts as well as your unborn baby. Avoid unpasteurized soft cheeses like feta, brie, blue cheese etc. Also avoid unpasteurized juice as well.

## Processed meats

A majority of processed meats such as lunch meats and hot dogs contain nitrates which play the role of a preservative. Nitrates can interfere with fertility. They can also cause a number of other health complications. Of late, most meats are being processed with lesser amounts of nitrates but still enough to hinder your fertility efforts.

## Caffeine

A small amount of caffeine is okay when you are trying to conceive but a large amount is not. Some studies have shown a connection between infertility and the consumption of large amounts of caffeine. Large amounts of caffeine have also been linked to miscarriage in some studies. It is recommended to limit your caffeine to 200 milligrams a day, the equivalent of one cup of coffee. This depends on the brew however. Don't forget that coffee isn't the only thing that contains caffeine. Caffeine is also found in carbonated drinks, chocolate, tea, and energy drinks.

## Sugar and simple carbs

In order to improve fertility, avoid simple carbohydrates,

refined sugars like high fructose corn syrup, and fructose. Even if a food label says "no sugar added" check the ingredients list. If fructose is on it, avoid it. Sugar and simple carbohydrates cause your body to produce insulin. Eventually your body gets use to functioning in an elevated insulin state. This temporary insulin resistance can decreases your fertility potential and proper ovarian function. It can also make your cervical mucus more acidic and less able to retain and protect sperm.

**High Mercury Fish**

High mercury fish are linked with infertility. They can also be harmful to your baby-to-be. Increase your chances of getting pregnant fast and avoid high mercury fish. The FDA recommends avoiding shark, king mackerel, swordfish, tilefish, and to eat only one serving (6 ounces) of solid white tuna per week.

## Trans Fats

Both you and your partner need to avoid all trans fats (hydrogenated or partially hydrogenated oils) found in fried or processed foods.

Read nutrition labels carefully in order to not overlook hidden trans fats. Choose foods with monounsaturated and polyunsaturated fats found in fatty fish, vegetable oils, and nuts.

Research suggests that trans fats have a huge effect on fertility health.

Reproductive hormonal pathways get blocked or altered in women by trans fats. This leads to numerous infertility problems.

For men, research has found that trans fats lower sperm count and quality.

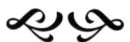

# Chapter 6

# Is It Possible To Conceive Naturally After 40?

There are many reasons why women are trying to conceive at forty or older. Some postpone pregnancy to advance their careers while others have been trying for a baby for a long time without any success.

Whatever the cause of their delay, the majority of these women can't help wondering whether it's too late for them to conceive in their forties.

The answer is simply, NO! You can still get pregnant at 40+! Yes, the chances of having a baby later in life are lower than when you were in your twenties and thirties but the fact remains that there are many happy, healthy babies born every year to women over forty.

*So, what are your chances of getting pregnant at this age?*

The truth is that it actually depends on how far along into your forties you are.

According to experts, your chances of conceiving are about twenty percent at forty and continue to dwindle to less than five percent by the time you hit your mid forties.

After you reach the age of forty five, it is highly possible that you may not have any chance of conceiving naturally.

Even so, there are many cases where women of this age have

conceived and delivered healthy babies.

According to health experts, the eggs of a woman begin to decline as early as fifteen years before she reaches menopause.

By forty five, your eggs will not only have reduced in quantity, but in quality as well. In fact, by the time you hit forty, your ovaries will probably start releasing eggs that have chromosomal abnormalities or structural problems. Such abnormalities have been known to raise the risk of birth defects and miscarriages

*What are your chances at fertility treatments?*

Fertility treatments such as ICSI and IVF have been getting better and better with time, and this has enhanced the chances of older women conceiving babies of their own or alternatively using frozen embryos or donor eggs.

Women who have attained the age of forty three and above have a minimal chance of conceiving using their own eggs and may have to consider using frozen embryos.

Women who conceive later in their forties and above are more likely to need extra care during pregnancy when compared to younger women.

In fact, whenever a pregnant woman of this age develops health problems, her doctor will likely classify her pregnancy as high risk.

While this might sound alarming, it only means that she should receive special care to ensure that her developing baby stays as healthy as possible. This is because such women are twice as likely to experience the following health conditions:

Pre-eclampsia

Gestational diabetes

High blood pressure

Placenta previa (low lying placenta)

Placenta abruption

Low-birth weight

Breech presentation (the baby's birth position is incorrect for delivery)

Caesarean section

Premature birth

If you have already reached the age of forty or higher and you and your partner have been having sex two or three times a week for a period of three months or more without conceiving, see your GP or healthcare provider to have some blood tests done. This will rule out any medical conditions that might be affecting your ability to conceive.

*Some of the conditions that might make it harder for you to conceive include the following:*

    Sexually transmitted disease/diseases

    Irregular periods

    Polycystic ovary syndrome

## Herbs that boost ovul[ation] and fertility

There are various homeopa[thic] remedies or herbs that are being used today to boost fertility. Experts warn however, that none have been proven to scientifically manipulate reproduction.

In spite of this, lots of women have claimed to benefit from them.

*Some of these herbs and supplements include:*

Chaste Tree Berry/Vitex

Dong Quai

False Unicorn Root

Wild Yam

FertilAid and Fertility Blend

Black Cohosh

Most of these fertility boosting herbs come from the Orient and can be purchased online or through herbal practitioners, acupuncturists or in Chinese clinics.

These herbs could very well be your answer to conception success.

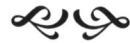

# Chapter 7

# Considering Different Ways to Get Pregnant

According to statistics, five out of six couples are able to conceive naturally. One out of six couples are not. These are the couples that have to consciously think about why they're not able to get pregnant and what they can do about it.

Typically, we associate 'getting pregnant' with sexual intercourse. Up until the 1900's this was the only way for couples to get pregnant.

Nowadays however there are two other options available that couples experiencing infertility can consider.

Intrauterine Insemination
(Low-tech approach)

In-Vitro-Fertilization
(High-tech approach)

## Intrauterine insemination

Intrauterine insemination is a method by which the sperm is deliberately delivered right to where the egg is waiting. In order to achieve this doctors collect sperm and then process it so that they are getting very clean sperm that is of the highest quality. They then put the clean processed sperm into a syringe and attach a catheter to it. Once the catheter is firmly attached, it is passed through the vagina and cervix into the uterine cavity. The sperm are deposited there.

In the uterine cavity, sperm have nowhere else to go but to the fallopian tubes. Some sperm may leak out but most remain. This makes it more likely that the sperm will reach the egg and fertilize it. This is not a high-tech, complicated method. It is quite straight forward. Even though couples that consider intrauterine insemination can get pregnant naturally, they have a higher chance of getting pregnant this way because there are so many more sperm available to reach the egg.

### In-Vitro-Fertilization

In-Vitro-Fertilization has been around since the late 1970's. It involves taking the eggs out of the body, bringing them into a laboratory and injecting the sperm straight into the egg or sprinkling the sperm on top of the egg. Once fertilized embryos are created, doctors watch them and then select the healthiest, best ones to transport through the cervix into the uterine cavity. The embryos will then continue the natural pregnancy process on their own by implanting themselves in the uterine cavity. This method is more high-tech than intrauterine insemination yet it acts as another way that couples can get pregnant.

## When to consider different ways of getting pregnant

The tips in this book will help you to get pregnant naturally. If you have been trying for quite some time to get pregnant and you've applied all the tips in this book and still haven't gotten pregnant then you have a choice. Either you can remain patient and keep trying to get pregnant naturally, or you can consider the alternate methods of getting pregnant.

It's only natural that your heart's desire might be to get pregnant naturally, but if you've exhausted all the reasons why it's not happening then you'll likely wonder how to know when it's time to consider the different alternatives.

*There are seven questions you can ask yourself that will help you with this:*

How many months have you tried to get pregnant but haven't?

How old are you?

Do you have any clues to suggest that there might be a certain problem that you should look into?

How important is it for you to get pregnant now?

What is your attitude toward getting pregnant?

Is your attitude "If it happens, it happens, if it doesn't, that's okay?"

Or is your attitude "It's really important to me to have a baby?"

Asking yourself these questions will help you to determine what the best option is for you.

If you decide to go the route of the alternate two methods, the good news is that your baby will be just as healthy and happy as if it was conceived naturally!

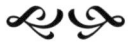

# **Conclusion**

Congratulations on finishing the book! Now you've got all the information you need to conceive for the first time!

Simply apply the advice provided in this book and you'll see results fast! Please don't delay because your precious little baby boy or girl can become a reality for you the sooner you get started.

I sincerely hope that you don't grow weary of applying the information in this book because I know first-hand how powerful it is. Please stick with it so that you too can achieve your dream of having a baby!

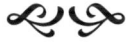

# About Paige Mathisen

*"Sharing what I've learned and what I love in books is my greatest joy!"*

I was always a curious child constantly exploring as much of my little world as possible. Everything was interesting to me!

As I explored, I jotted down notes on what I was learning and I constantly asked questions that I was determined to find answers for.

My curiosity habit stayed with me as I grew and in college I began turning my notes into mini-books. Well, actually, they were more like manuscripts coiled and bound at my local office supply store.

I ran little seminars on topics I was interested in and sold my manuscripts to anyone that was interested in purchasing them. Surprisingly, I sold quite a few!

Years later with the rise of self-publishing, I began turning my book writing, curiosity habit, into an actual business.

Now, my little world has gotten bigger as I'm married and have two beautiful children ...and a golden retriever! I'm blessed to be able to write every day on a wide variety of topics that I'm completely passionate about!

I put my heart and soul into every book I write and my biggest hope is that I can help you understand whatever it is that you are seeking answers for.

My belief is that great books don't have to be expensive, nor do they have to be particularly long.

That's why I write shorter books that are relatively inexpensive. I do my best to give you the best "bang for your buck" by over-delivering and giving you all the necessary information you need on a specific topic.

Thank you in advance for allowing me to share my passion and experience with you!

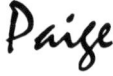

Made in the USA
Middletown, DE
04 December 2015